The Adventures of Sophie Bean

The Pond Hockey Challenge

written by
Kathryn Yevchak with Lynn Omslaer

illustrated by
Judith Pfeiffer

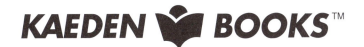

KAEDEN BOOKS™

For my family.
—Kathy

Title: The Adventures of Sophie Bean: The Pond Hockey Challenge
Copyright © 2008 Kaeden Corporation
Author: Kathryn Yevchak with Lynn Omslaer
Illustrator: Judith Pfeiffer

ISBN: 978-1-57874-428-2

Published by:
   Kaeden Corporation
   P.O. Box 16190
   Rocky River, Ohio 44116
   1-800-890-7323
   www.kaeden.com

Printed in Canada

10 9 8 7 6 5 4 3 2 1

Contents

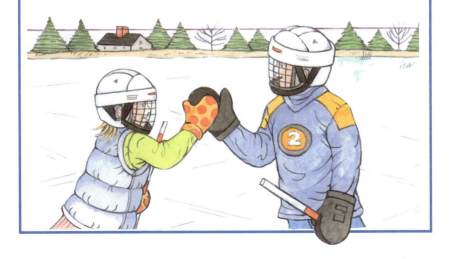

—1—

Finally Frozen

"Time for some ice skating!" Aunt Lynn shouted.

It was wintertime, and the large pond in the backyard of Ryan and Parker's house was frozen solid. Sophie Bean and her twin cousins, Ryan and Parker, were getting ready to ice skate.

"Remember, I don't want anyone ice skating unless an adult is out here with you," said Aunt Lynn.

"We know, we know," said Parker. Ryan and Parker were already

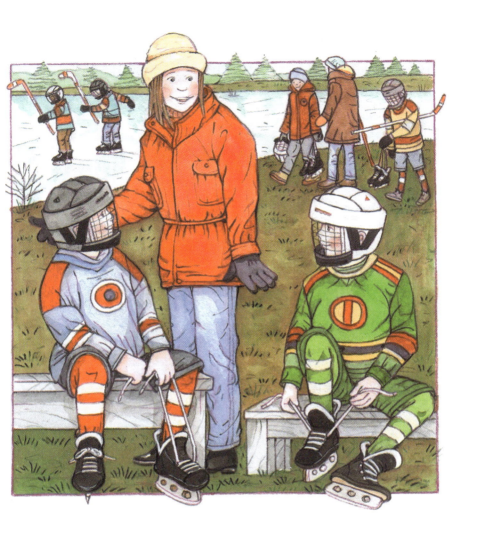

tightening the laces on their ice
skates so they could set up the goal
nets and start playing ice hockey. The
neighborhood boys and some of their
moms were arriving for the game.

Sophie Bean sat on the bench near the edge of the frozen pond looking concerned. She looked at the hand-me-down, black ice hockey skates she had from Ryan and thought that nice, white figure skates would look much better with her pink sweatpants. Sophie Bean looked out at the ice again. There was no railing to hold on to like at the indoor ice skating rink.

"Hurry up, Sophie Bean. You can be goalie," said Parker as he put on his helmet.

"Come on, Sophie Bean, you don't want to be the most slippery bean again like last year, do you?" asked Ryan with a grin.

Sophie Bean sighed. How was she ever going to be a hockey goalie when she didn't know the first thing about playing ice hockey and she could barely skate without holding on to a railing?

"I think I'm just going to watch today," said Sophie Bean from the bench.

"Sophie Bean, Sophie Bean, the most slippery bean we've ever seen!" chanted Ryan and Parker.

She sat and watched as Ryan, Parker and a couple of their neighborhood friends – all boys – finished setting up the goal nets.

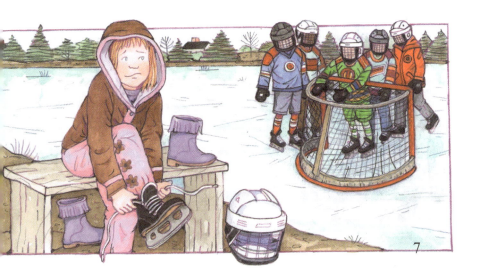

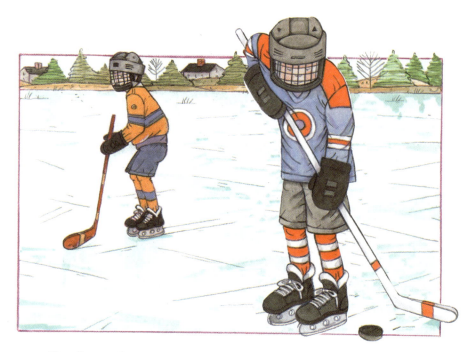

Before long, the game began and Ryan was gliding quickly across the ice and scoring a goal.

"Yes!" Ryan cheered holding his hockey stick up in the air. "Hat trick, here I come!"

Sophie Bean wondered what in the world a hat trick could be when everyone was wearing helmets.

"It's going to be a long winter," said Sophie Bean with a sigh.

—2—

Double Blades No More

Sophie Bean looked up from the bench where she was still sitting and saw Mommy walking down toward the pond. Last winter, Sophie Bean had double-bladed ice skates and had been able to skate holding Mommy's hand or clinging to the railing at the indoor ice rink. She slipped all over the place and got teased for it all winter long by her two older cousins, Ryan and Parker.

This year, the double-bladed skates no longer fit her.

"Looks like you are going to have to learn on regular ice skates this year," said Mommy. She knelt down and tightened the laces on Sophie Bean's skates. "Okay, Sophie Bean, I'll help you onto the ice. Come on, you can do it!"

"Okay, I'll try," said Sophie Bean, determined not to let Ryan and Parker's teasing stop her.

Mommy walked Sophie Bean out onto the ice. But suddenly, Mommy was gone, off to catch their dog, Cody, who was chasing a squirrel and getting too close to the street.

"Cody! Get back here!" Mommy shouted. "Sophie Bean, I'll be right back!"

But it was too late, Sophie Bean's legs started to spread wider and wider

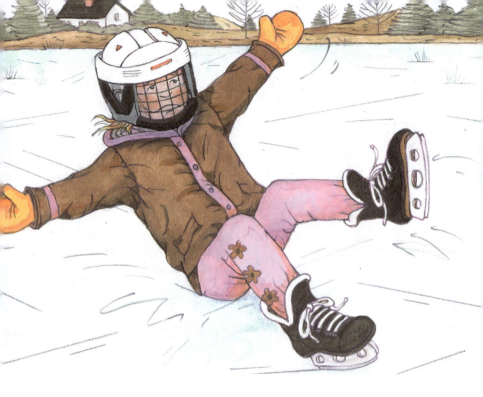

apart as if she was doing a split in gymnastics class. Ryan, Parker and all of their friends stopped skating and watched as her skates grew farther and farther apart, until SPLAT, down onto the ice went Sophie Bean.

"Sophie Bean, Sophie Bean the most slippery bean we've ever seen!" sang Ryan. The boys giggled and went back to their hockey game.

Sophie Bean crawled over to the edge of the pond and sat on the cold, hard ground as she untied her skates and pulled them off.

"I'm going to have some hot chocolate," said Sophie Bean. She walked in her pink and purple polka-dotted socks back up to Aunt Lynn's house.

"What's the matter Sophie Bean? Why aren't you skating?" asked Aunt Lynn as Sophie Bean came inside.

"I can't skate! The double blades don't fit me anymore and there's no railing and Mommy wasn't out there to hold my hand because Cody ran off and Ryan and Parker keep laughing at me!" cried Sophie Bean.

Mommy came in with Cody and overheard what Sophie Bean was saying.

"It's okay, sweetie, before long you'll be out there skating with your silly cousins. You'll see," said Mommy with a hug around Sophie Bean's shoulders. "Now, there's nothing a little hot chocolate can't cure."

Sophie Bean sat by Aunt Lynn's fireplace warming up, waiting for the hot chocolate to cool off so she wouldn't burn her tongue and watching Ryan and Parker through the big picture window as they skated smoothly around the ice.

"I just have to figure out a way to get on that ice," said Sophie Bean.

—3—

A Big Bowl of Milk

The next week, Sophie Bean's older cousin Justin came home from college for his winter break. Sophie Bean called him on the telephone. She knew that before Justin left for college, he had played on his high school's ice hockey team.

"Justin, you won't believe it. Ryan and Parker won't stop teasing me about my ice skating. I can't help it if the ice is slippery!" said Sophie Bean.

"Oh, don't worry about Ryan and Parker. When they were little, I taught them how to ice skate. They used to slip and slide all over the place too."

"Really?" asked Sophie Bean.

"Really. How about we head over to the ice rink by your house tomorrow? I'll give you some pointers," said Justin.

"Great! I can't wait," said Sophie Bean.

Sophie Bean hung up the phone feeling a little bit better.

Bright and early the next morning, Justin picked up Sophie Bean at her house.

"Remember, stay with Justin the whole time," called Mommy from the front door as Sophie Bean and Justin left for the ice rink.

Before she knew it, they were at the ice rink and Justin was helping her tighten up the laces on her ice skates and buckle her helmet.

Sophie Bean clung to Justin's hand as they stepped out onto the ice.

"What if I fall?" asked Sophie Bean, looking up at Justin with fear in her eyes.

"Don't worry, everyone falls," said Justin. "It's like falling into a big bowl of milk," he added.

"A big bowl of milk?" Sophie Bean

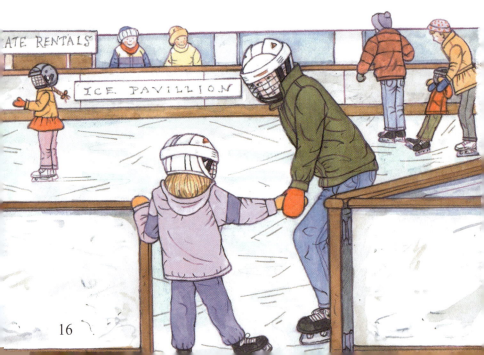

thought that the hard ice hitting her bottom wouldn't feel anything like splashing into a bowl of milk.

"Well, maybe not exactly, but that's what my dad used to tell me when I was little," said Justin with a grin.

With one hand, Sophie Bean clung to Justin's hand and with her other hand, she held on to the wall of the ice rink.

"Remember, there's no wall at the pond. You are going to have to let go. Just pretend you are marching on the ice. Hut, two, three, four," said Justin as he let go of her hand and pretended to march on the ice.

All of a sudden, as he turned around to face Sophie Bean, the blade of Justin's ice skate hit a small hole in the ice. SPLAT! Justin's feet flew out from underneath him and he landed flat on his back.

"Justin! Are you okay?" cried Sophie Bean.

Justin looked up slowly, "See, I told you. Everyone falls."

Sophie Bean giggled, let go of the wall and began marching toward Justin as he stood up from his fall.

All afternoon, Justin and Sophie Bean practiced marching on the ice.

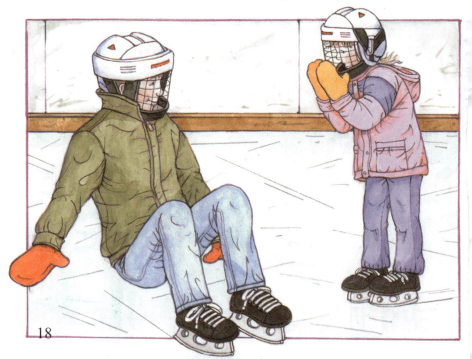

Then, they moved on to marching and gliding.

"March, march, glide, glide. That's it! You've got it!" said Justin. "See, you're not a slippery little bean anymore. You can do it!"

Almost as soon as the words came out of Justin's mouth, Sophie Bean's feet slid out from under her and SPLAT, down on the ice she went. Sophie Bean felt her eyes start to fill with tears.

"Now that you're down there, let's practice getting up," said Justin.

He talked her through it: "That's it … just kneel on both knees with your hands on the ice, next to your knees. Now, lift one knee up and then the other. Steady yourself with your hands on the ice. Then stretch your arms out for balance and slowly stand up. Great!"

At the end of the day, Sophie Bean was exhausted and hungry.

"Can we go get a snack now?" asked Sophie Bean.

They headed up to the snack bar and bought two hot pretzels.

"Justin, do you know what a hat trick is?" asked Sophie Bean.

"A hat trick is when one player scores three goals during an ice hockey game," explained Justin.

"So that's what Ryan meant," said Sophie Bean.

After their long day of practice, Sophie Bean felt like she was almost ready to skate on the pond by herself.

—4—

The Rules of Hockey

For the rest of the time that Justin was home from college, he took Sophie Bean ice skating almost every day. A couple of times, he brought his brothers, Connor and Jack.

"Sophie Bean, we've all been playing ice hockey for years. We can teach you how to play," said Connor.

Before long, Sophie Bean was learning all kinds of things she'd never heard of before. Justin, Connor and Jack showed her the correct way to hold her hockey stick, how to pass the hockey puck and how to shoot at the goal.

Sophie Bean also had to learn all of the rules of the game.

"Make sure you don't check any of the other players. That means you can't push them really hard," explained Jack. "I know that sometimes you might want to push Parker, but it's against the rules."

"And no slashing or hitting the other players' legs with your hockey stick like this," Connor added, as he pretended to go after Jack with his stick.

"Penalty!" shouted Jack as he skated away from Connor.

"Cut it out, guys! We're supposed to be helping Sophie Bean," reminded Justin.

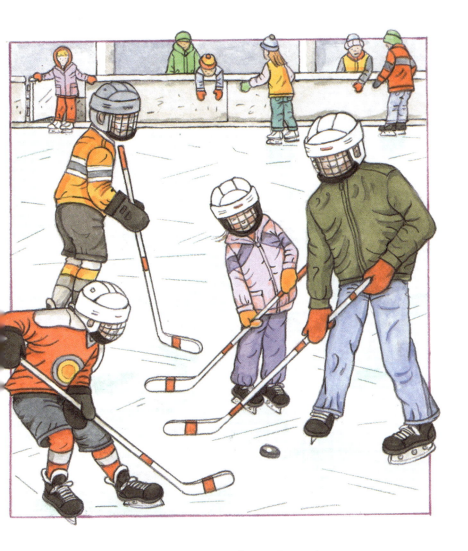

Then, it was time for Justin to go back to college. Connor and Jack lived too far away to skate every day with Sophie Bean.

She was now on her own.

—5—

The Challenge Is On

"Sophie Bean, come on, we'll be late! We have to leave now to make it for the start of the game!" called Mommy.

The cousins were all heading to the men's ice hockey game at the college in the next town.

Sophie Bean came downstairs in a pink dress, tights and sparkly red shoes.

"You can't wear that to a hockey game! You'll freeze!" laughed Ryan.

"Then you would be Sophie Bean, Sophie Bean, the chilliest bean we've

ever seen," said Parker, pretending to
shiver and rub his arms.

"But I want to wear a dress!"
pleaded Sophie Bean to Mommy.

"Oh, alright, you don't have time to
change. Let's just grab an extra
blanket for you," said Mommy.

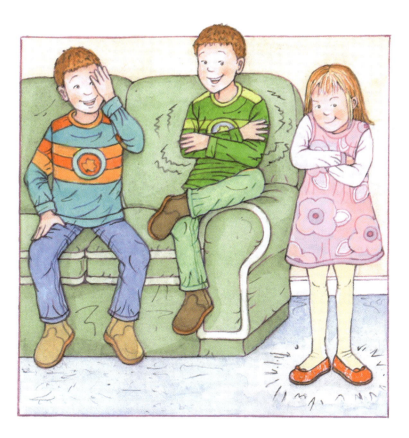

At the hockey game, the three cousins were cheering for the green team because green was Parker's favorite color. Parker was, of course, dressed in head-to-toe green, right down to his socks.

During the first intermission, about ten spectators were chosen to play musical chairs right on the ice. They were sliding all over the place because they were still wearing their regular shoes on the ice.

"Look, Sophie Bean, they are as slippery as you are on the ice!" said Ryan.

"You just wait, Ryan, I'll show you what a good ice skater I am now!" said Sophie Bean.

"Oh, really? I can't wait to see it. Come over in the morning, we're playing hockey again," said Ryan.

That night, Sophie Bean could
barely sleep. All she could think about
was the hockey game at Ryan and
Parker's pond in the morning. She
crawled out of bed and into Mommy's
room.

"Mommy, I can't sleep. What if I
slide all over the ice again?" asked
Sophie Bean.

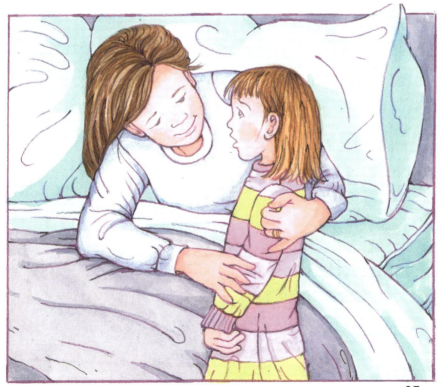

"Oh, sweetie, you will be fine. Just remember everything that Justin taught you," said Mommy as she walked Sophie Bean back to her bed. "Now, get some sleep."

Over and over, Sophie Bean thought about all of the things Justin, Connor and Jack had taught her.

"March, march, glide, glide. I can do it!" thought Sophie Bean as she finally drifted off to sleep and dreamed not about playing hockey, but about twirling and spinning on the ice like a graceful figure skater.

—6—

Time to Prove It

The next morning, Sophie Bean came downstairs wearing her favorite pink, twirly corduroy skirt.

"Sophie Bean, you can't wear that for the hockey game!" said Mommy. "Go put on some pants!"

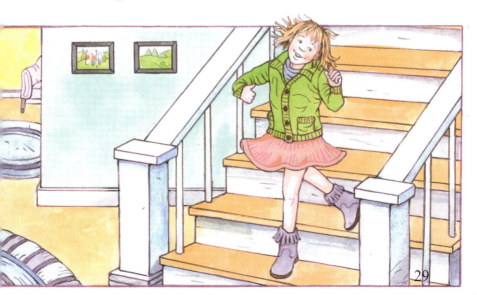

"But, Mommy, please!" pleaded Sophie Bean.

"Well … okay, but put some leggings on underneath the skirt," said Mommy.

When they finally arrived at Aunt Lynn's house for the big game, all of the neighborhood boys were already there setting up the goal nets.

"Why are you wearing a skirt?" Parker asked Sophie Bean. He shrugged and said, "Girls are so weird!"

"Hey, Sophie Bean, we've been waiting for you. Let's see if you can really skate," challenged Ryan.

Mommy helped Sophie Bean lace up her ice skates. Then Mommy held Sophie Bean's hand as she stepped onto the ice.

"You don't have to hold on to me, Mommy. I can do it by myself," said Sophie Bean.

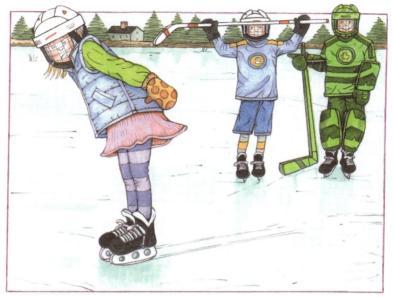

Ryan and Parker watched Sophie Bean closely. They were sure that she would be sliding all over the place in no time.

March, march, glide, glide … Sophie Bean was gliding on the ice! She was a little wobbly, but at least she wasn't falling down.

"See, Ryan, I told you I could do it! I'm not the most slippery bean anymore!" said Sophie Bean looking triumphant.

"Ryan, let Sophie Bean play on your team today," ordered Mommy.

"Okay, okay," Ryan agreed.

The game started and Sophie Bean worked very hard at not falling and remembering all of the hockey rules at the same time.

Parker was playing goalie for the other team. Of course, his entire outfit was green, including his hockey stick, gloves, goalie pads and elaborately decorated green goalie helmet.

The boys zoomed all around Sophie Bean expertly passing the hockey puck back and forth. Before long, Ryan had scored a goal. And then another!

"Oh, man!" said Parker, disappointed that he had not stopped the puck.

"That's two goals for Ryan. He's close to a hat trick," said Sophie Bean as she tried desperately to remain steady on the ice.

All of a sudden, the hockey puck was coming right towards her. Sophie Bean started to panic, but then, she just kept remembering all of the things she had learned from Justin. She set the hockey stick on the ice in front of her and SLAM ... she stopped the puck! The boys from the other team were getting closer. Parker was looking at her through the green goalie mask, ready to stop her shot. Sophie Bean pulled the hockey stick back and with all of her might, shot the puck towards the goal. Parker went diving down to the left.

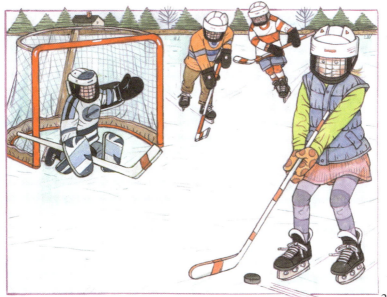

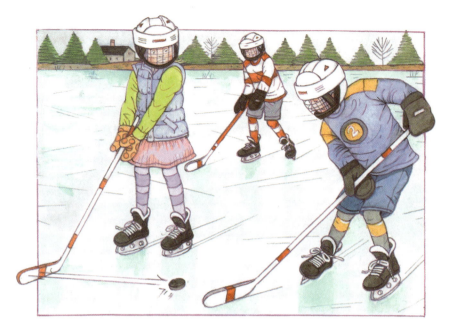

"Oh, no," thought Sophie Bean. The puck sputtered and bounced a little and looked like it was going to miss the goal.

But then, at the last minute, Ryan came speeding up and scooped the puck up with his stick and shot it into the upper right-hand corner of the net.

Parker saw what was happening, but it was too late. He tried to stand up and reach for the puck, but slipped and landed on the ice.

"Score!" shouted Ryan. It was Ryan's third goal of the game.

"YES! You did it, Ryan! Hat trick!" Sophie Bean shouted.

Mommy and Aunt Lynn were cheering from the side of the pond. Even Cody was barking his approval.

Parker was lying on the ice looking up at them still not believing that the puck went into the goal.

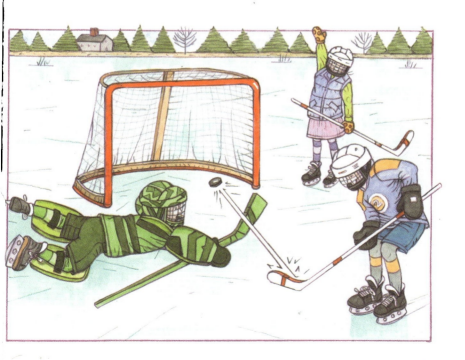

"It looks like you're the most slippery one now, Parker!" said Sophie Bean with a big grin on her face.

"Nice assist, Sophie Bean," said Ryan.

Ryan gave Sophie Bean a big high-five and together they skated back to the center of the pond to set up for the next face-off.

"You can be on my team anytime," Ryan said.

Sophie Bean grinned and couldn't wait to call Justin and tell him the good news. Sophie Bean was now a hockey player.

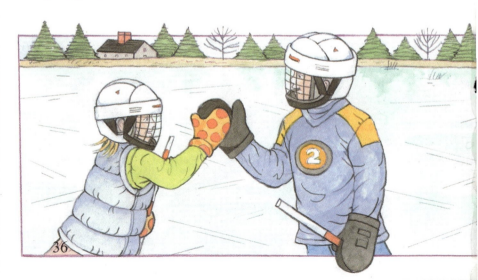